I0118566

YOGA TRANSFORMATIONS
MINDFUL NEW BEGINNINGS

by

Cynthia Lynne, MFCT
Lifeforce© Yoga Therapist

Copyright @ 2013 :

Cynthia Naughton, M.A., MFCT, Counseling & Coaching

P.O. Box 266, Santa Barbara, CA   93102

ISBN 13 : 978 0984727797 :   ISBN 10 : 0984727795

Women's Health & Fitness : Therapeutic Yoga : Self Help

An Invitation for you....

Begin again anew

A Mindful Reprieve : Beyond Burn Out Model

BEYOND SICK AND TIRED

By Cynthia Lynne, Lifeforce© Yoga Therapist   Copyright 2013

ARE YOU A HIGH ACHIEVER SUFFERING FROM STRESS OVERLOAD?

According to the American Psychological Association, American Institute of Stress 2013 Study:

77% of Americans report they suffer physically over their stress – fatigue, headaches, muscle tension

73% of Americans suffer psychological distress over their stress, including nervousness, irritability, depression and poor motivation

48% of Americans say they lie awake at night over their stress

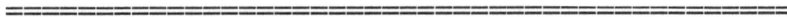

==

When does a high achiever become an overachiever bordering on burn out?

Are you one of these people?

"People who are under chronic stress are more likely to gain weight and to smoke, and are less likely to sleep well or exercise," which increases their risk for cardiovascular disease, diabetes, stroke , obesity and other serious medical diseases. "

IMPOSSIBLE BINDS

==

What do many people do to solve their stressed out state of overload?

They create more problems by what they perceive is a "solution" to the brain and body in stress overdrive...like...

Beat themselves into a dieting or exercise program they hate...

Berate themselves for failing to accomplish their goals...

Push themselves even harder to do what now has become impossible..

Sound familiar?

==

MINDFUL INQUIRY : Ask without judging

Where do you draw the line on pursuits of futility and frustration?

What do you say no to?

When do you draw the line?

Before burn out?
Or is burn out your body's way of drawing the line *for you?*

STOP!

DO SOMETHING DIFFERENT!

PAUSE.

REFLECT…on the possibilities of MINDFULNESS….

What do millions of yogis know that you most need to transform your life?

BECOME MINDFUL IN YOUR DAILY HABITS

By *doing* daily yoga habits, you will become acquainted with the power of *being*.

Soon you'll understand how being can help you go with the flow of transformative change….

Doing daily yoga will help you learn how to *be*.

Choose simple mindful daily practices to balance body, brain and chemistry.
This can change how you feel with what you choose.

Simple choices in what you eat and how you move can make all the difference for the biochemistry of the body and brain.

Begin with a mindful review.
Step back. Breathe.

Reflect upon your options.

Become mindful through the process of mindful inquiry. Ask a meaningful question. Simply reflect upon the possibilities that arise from meaning.

Consider the possibility of mindfulness.

What would happen if you were to become mindful in thought, word and deed?

FREEDOM OF CHOICE

==

Yes, you are free to choose your particular brand of craziness.

If you truly believe burning the candle at both ends is your path to success, you are free to choose.

Then again, you are free to choose something different…aren't you?

What if you were to choose to STOP and Hit the "RESET" button?

What would immediately change for you if you make this choice?

Why not….?
Begin again anew.

==

By Cynthia Lynne, Lifeforce© Yoga Therapist   Copyright 2013

MINDFUL PURSUITS OF POSSIBILITY

You could choose to…

Let go of pushing your self to DO more.

You could choose to….

Let go of over do-do-doing to reach an imaginary state of nirvana.

You could choose to become mindful in your daily pursuits, couldn't you?

THE FREEDOM TO BE …

You *could choose* to stop doing and start **being**.

Do being for a change.

Say what? How do you <u>do</u> being?

Simple.

Do mindful daily practices – like the ones you'll learn in this guide.

Let your body expand your mind into clarity, insight and a laser focus on what is possible…

Make possible the impossible…
Let go of impossible binds…

Take a leap of faith….

SIGNS OF CHRONIC STRESS OVERLOAD

===

How many "yes" answers to you have to the following questions:

1.Do you often feel overworked pressured or deadlined?

2. Do you have problems with feeling "uptight" and "edgy"

3. Does your body tend to feel stiff or tense or achy?

4. Are you easily upset, frustrated or snappy under pressure?

5. Do you often feel overwhelmed?

6. Do you feel weak or shaky at times?

7. Do you sensitive to bright light, noise or chemical fumes?

8. Do you feel significantly worse if you skip meals or go too long without eating?

9. Do you use tobacco, alcohol, food or drugs to relax, self soothe or calm down?

10. Do you suffer from depression or mood swings?

AN EPIDEMIC OF "STRESSED OUT"

Unhappy with your results?   You *are not* alone!

==

THE STATISTICS :

Only 37% of Americans say they do a very good job at managing their stress.

  48% reported they overeat over their stress
  39% reported skipping meals over their stress

Only 33% say they were very good at being physically active.
     *American Psychological Association 2013

==

WHAT IF .....?

What if you ….

Focus on the Solution to the Problem of Stress Overload :

Let go of Solving a Problem with a Problem (a diet, a harsh dose of "more of the same")

Focus on Shifting Burn Out Beliefs that set you up to stress out over doing more to solve the problem of feeling overwhelmed.

Allow your body to heal your mind….

By Cynthia Lynne, Lifeforce© Yoga Therapist   Copyright 2013

Discover the power of mindfulness to...*get twice as much done in half the time...*

Imagine...*if you, too, could* do *less and*

be more and

get twice as much done

in half the time?

YOGA TRANSFORMATIONS
A MINDFUL NEW BEGINNING

Your Mindful Guide ....

TABLE OF CONTENTS :

TABLE OF CONTENTS : continued

By Cynthia Lynne, Lifeforce© Yoga Therapist   Copyright 2013

TABLE OF CONTENTS : continued

A RADICAL SHIFT IN THINKING AND CHOOSING

The radical shift begins with a choice to let go.

Let go of fooling yourself into believing what you're doing now is working for you.

Admit you have become your own worst enemy.
The beliefs you believe in are making you sick and tired.

Surrender to your higher wisdom.
The wisdom hidden within.

Stop doing what you've been doing.
Become present to the power of stillness.

Slow down to find your center of calm strength.

It resides within….
Your center of innate wisdom.

Begin now, the journey of true discovery…

Quiet the mind to discover the fire that burns within..

Discover the eternal life truths that lift you into infinite possibilities….

By Cynthia Lynne, Lifeforce© Yoga Therapist   Copyright 2013

Get Yoga Fit in Body, Mind & Spirit

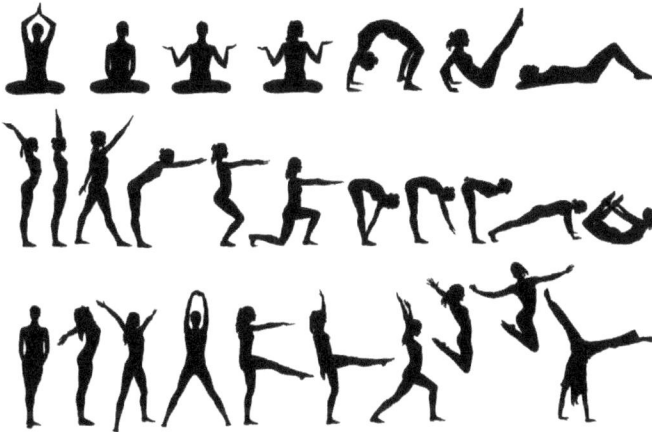

Yogis realized thousands of years ago that changing dysfunctional habits is largely a matter of the mind.
It was the mind that was the yogi's most interesting subject of study. The true intention of a daily yoga practice was to access this "enlightened awareness" through taming the fluctuations of the mind.

From *Yoga as Medicine* By T. McCall, M.D.

===

WHAT IS MINDFULNESS?

Mindfulness is a centuries old principle and practice originating in the Middle East.

Mindfulness is a practice and a presence, a discipline that cultivates greater awareness to the innate wisdom of the body, mind and human spirit.

Mindfulness is being fully embodied in the present moment in time.

Mindfulness is… a powerful state of mind and body.

*Mindfulness is…*a keen state of awareness in mind and body

Mindfulness is …. an attitude

Mindfulness is… a transformational mind/body tool

THE HEALING POWER OF MINDFULNESS MEDICINE FOR THE MIND AND BODY

Studies conducted over the past twenty five years indicates mindfulness meditation can **decrease depression, relieve anxiety, reduce fatigue, increase tolerance to stress, slow the heart rate** and **decrease blood pressure; strengthen the body's immune system** and **decrease physical pain.**

(Baer 2003, Baer, Fischer & Hass, 2005a, Brown, Ryan and Creswell 2007; Kabat-Zinn, 1990)

A MINDFUL INVITATION…..

Would you be willing to break out of the comfort zone of your present habits to begin a mindful daily practice instead?

What would it take for you to be all in for mindfulness?

What would stop you from being all in for mindfulness?

===

Change begins here and now.

Choose mindfulness.

Begin with a Mindful New Beginning....

COURTING RESILIENCE THROUGH RELAXATION

You could choose to court your body's relaxation response through a daily yoga practice, couldn't you?

You could *choose* to take ten minutes to chill out rather than spin out on a daily basis, couldn't you?

IMAGINE ....

Relaxing into calm strength

Healing your burnt out body, mind and spirit

Releasing mindsets and burn out beliefs

Restoring vitality

Being your best

The power of a mindful mind, body and spirit......

What if you could accomplish twice as much in half the time?

What if you, too, would – just like others before you have….

What would stop you from choosing mindfulness?

Would you begin now…if you are free to choose?

What could a daily yoga practice do for you?

Discover the power of yoga to create purposeful practices to inspire and motivate you in ways you haven't yet thought possible....

Build New Neural Pathways :
If you could build mental strength and fitness with a simple daily yoga practice, why not help your brain help you change from the inside out?

Rebalance Hormone Levels :
If a daily yoga practice could help you balance your hormones so you feel better, think better and carry less "stress weight," would you choose ten minutes a day to do yoga?

Replenish Healthy Mood Chemicals :
If essential mood chemicals are depleted by chronic stress, couldn't daily meditations and mantras help your mind release healthy endorphins to improve your mood?

Relax the Emotional Body & Mind :
If daily yoga practices helps the emotional body avoid a build up of muscular tension and tightness, would you find ten minutes in your day to spend time in your "zen zone?"

Yoga is a daily practice that encourages the brain to create new neural pathways

JUST SAY "OMMMMM"…..

After the tsunami ripped through Southeast Asia in 2004 came a tidal wave of psychic devastation. The depression and posttraumatic <u>stress</u> that ravaged many residents of coastal villages from India to Indonesia provided a living laboratory for testing the most powerful cures available.

What wound up providing the best help to some of the most afflicted refugees?

Yoga.

As a professor of <u>psychiatry</u> at New York Medical College who studies the effects of yoga on posttraumatic stress, Patricia Gerbarg seized the opportunity to test whether it could help tsunami survivors in India. To one group of 60 victims she gave a four-day yoga breathing course. Another group of 60 survivors was given the yoga course along with psychological counseling. A third group served as controls.

All the yoga users experienced a huge drop in scores for posttraumatic stress disorder and depression after just four days. And the effect was so persistent that Gerbarg and her <u>team</u> introduced yoga to those in the control group too. Counseling provided no added benefits over the yoga training alone.

While some forms of yoga have long been shown to reduce hypertension, cholesterol levels, and other signs of physiological stress, the effects of the ancient practice on psychological stress have been less studied.   But a slew of research published in peer-reviewed journals in the U.S., Europe, and India is documenting *the ability of yoga to decrease mood disturbance, reduce psychic stress and anxiety, and reduce <u>PTSD</u> symptoms.*

Positive benefits of yoga breath practice have been seen within days of initiating instruction, and have been documented up to six months after a course of yoga training.

PROFOUND SHIFTS IN EMOTIONAL STATES

Gerbarg's studies *have found that yogic breathing physiologically affects the nervous system to produce profound changes in emotional states.*

Deep yogic breath acts on the vagus nerve—the "rest and digest" response or calming pathway of the autonomic nervous system that extends from <u>brain</u> stem to abdomen.

When the vagus nerve is activated, it helps to *automatically slow down breathing* and *heart rate* and increases intestinal activity. It not only carries signals from brain to body but ferries signals from the body back to the brain.

Science shows how our breathing pattern changes with emotional reactions to things," Gerbarg says.

"...when you change your breathing pattern, you can change your emotions."

From *Yoga as Medicine* By T. McCall, M.D.

Ancient yogis practiced yoga daily to create new habits or what they called "samskaras." Today's scientist would call these new neural pathways.

Samskaras are daily habits of action and thought that create new disciplines as well as new awarenesses.

Yogis believed that everytime you do or think something, you increase the likelihood that you will do or think it again. This is true of both desirable and undesirable thoughts and actions

===

Ancient yogis manipulated the body in every way they could think of...experimented with various techniques for channeling the breath...and created a series of postures designed to **systematically work every part of the body and create awareness where there was none."**

===

The yogic model of daily practice both creates new neural pathways and strengthens these pathways through repetition. Daily practice isn't about getting it perfect – but about deepening the grooves of new neural pathways through consistency and repetition.

===

If yoga could heal post traumatic stress, could a daily yoga practice heal burn out?

Could a daily yoga practice help you build calm strength that would heal your body, mind and troubled spirit?

Could a daily yoga practice be exactly the tool needed build emotional resilience – an essential "stress buster?"

By Cynthia Lynne, Lifeforce© Yoga Therapist   Copyright 2013

Why not do what ancient yogis did?

Use the power of a daily yoga practice to transform body and mind

Work with the forces of change ….
Let go of forcing change…

See what a difference aligning with body and mind can make in your outcomes…

What would stop you from choosing mindfulness?

So let's begin now….

TEN MINDFUL MOMENTS TO BEGIN

Is a part of your mind thinking "I don't have time for a daily practice. I'm too busy to make time for anything else!"

What if it takes less time than you presently believe to begin a daily yoga practice?

What if it only takes ten minutes to start...

==

Where could you find ten minutes to begin again anew?

Where could you subtract a "doing" to add in a "being" moment?

==

BEGIN AGAIN ANEW...
TAKE TEN MINDFUL MOMENTS

Ten minutes. Such a small slice of time to reset ....

If time is a pie, how many time slices do you have available to you in the entire pie?

How much of a slice is ten minutes?

What if you could slice out a tiny sliver of time to begin satisfy your body's need to restore and rebalance?

How many slices would remain?

=======================================

The Ten Minutes Challenge : Track your Time : One Day in Time

Set an intention to track all of the time you spend beginning tomorrow. Use a notepad and write things like *"breakfast 1 minute; stretching; 2 minutes; checking wardrobe 5 minutes; driving to work; 10 minutes"*

   (1) How many minutes a day you stand in line?

   (2) How many minutes a day are you idling on hold? Sitting in traffic? Fiddling with a gadget of some sort?

   (3) How many minutes a day do you scroll through e-mails that don't matter, watch television that you don't care about or carry on a conversation that wastes time and energy?

Total the Numbers:
At the end of the day add up all of your totals and rate them accordingly:
1: high value
2: modest value
3: minimal value
4: waste of time, energy & resources
5. drain of time, energy & resources

MINDFUL REVIEW :

MINDFUL REVIEW : Review the results and notice your thoughts & feelings about what you've discovered. No judgment – simple awareness.

MINDFUL INQUIRY :   Ask a Meaningful Question: the key to change is an essential shift in self awareness; without meaningful reflection or mindful inquiry, you are destined to repeat old patterns of thought and habit.

What inspires me about my answers?

What do I wish to change?

How could I make this change if I chose to change?

Seize the Moment : Begin Now....

Why does our brain make it so complicated?

Why do we buy into the belief that we have to make a project out of exercise or fitness?

Why do we believe exercise has to be a unique form of torture or punishment for dieting sins not yet committed?

The mind can convince us into believing fictions we create to avoid the discomfort of change.

Watch your mind as it convinces you into resisting change...

What if you were to move past the resistance into a powerful flow of energy like water rushing past rocks?

What if you were simply to seize the moment and breathe deeply into your body until you feel your belly move into rhythm and expand?

Begin to move into your day before you even fully awaken to the possibility of your breath becoming one with your body.

What is the rhythm of your breath that awakens you into your day with energy, clarity and excitement?

Stretch into your body. Breathe into your stretch. Notice what you notice about how it feels to move.

What movement helps your body feel good?

Daily Yoga Practice Intention: Take Ten for Yoga:

Start with a simple intention to take ten minutes a day for yoga.

Begin the day with yoga.
End the day with yoga.

Take a ten minute break somewhere in your day.

Just take ten for yoga.

Begin to experience the power of a consistent yoga practice.

Dedicate time and space for your body to discover its unique rhythm and movement.

Let yoga guide you into the rhythm and movement that suits your body just right.

Wake up to the intention of breathing into your body and awareness of the rhythm of your breath.

Take time to listen to the song of body and breath uniting as one….
…..before you open your eyes to the morning light…

SIMPLE MINDFUL PRACTICE : AWAKEN TO YOGA

Wake up to the intention of breathing deeply into your body until you feel the rhythm of your breath.

Simply breathe. Slowly. Smoothly. Deeply.

Take time to listen to the song of body and breath uniting as one….before you open your eyes to the morning light…

Inhale deeply into your nostrils; pause before you expand deeply into your lungs : slowly exhale and relax deeply into the expanding of your breath into your belly.

Breathe deeply to awaken the body gently with breath…

Relax as you release into the center of your body and breathe into the energy of awakening.

Draw the source of your energy from deep within the body. Breathe – slowly, smoothly and deeply into your body.

Feel your belly rise and fall with the rhythm of your breath.

Focus on drawing your belly into your backbone as you exhale, deeply and fully.

Pause as you feel the power of belly to back. Relax into the sensations.

Inhale again. Relax. Release.

Simple to start.

Just get started…!

By Cynthia Lynne, Lifeforce© Yoga Therapist   Copyright 2013

Where can you find ten minutes to begin again anew?

Awaken to Joy & Inspired Purpose

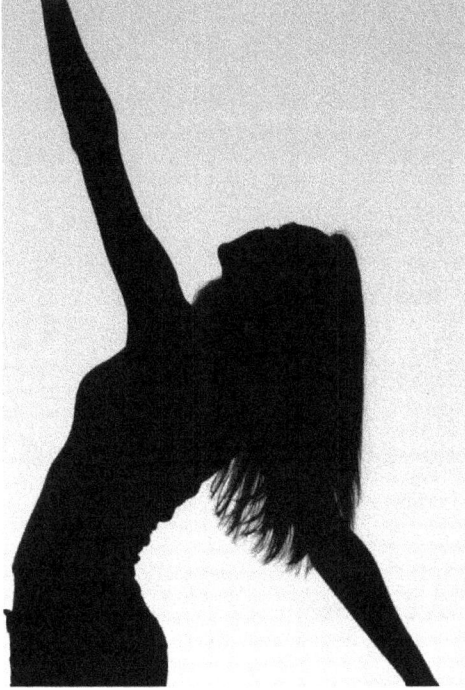

Move into action!
Stand up!
Stretch your arms out!
Reach up!

Breathe deep into the center of your body!
Draw circles with your arms and feel warmth of energy rising into your chest.

Breathe again.
Release into energy moving through your body into your limbs.

Breathe deeply into your belly center.
Move past the resistance, feel the power of simply movement to energize your body.

Let yoga move you past the impasse.
Just move!

By Cynthia Lynne, Lifeforce© Yoga Therapist   Copyright 2013

JUST BREATHE

Inhale deeply into your nostrils; pause before you exhale and relax deeply into the expanding of your breath.

Breathe deeply to awaken the body gently with breath…

Relax as you release into the center of your body and breathe into the energy of awakening.

Draw the source of your energy from deep within the body. Breathe – slowly, smoothly and deeply into your body.

Feel your belly rise and fall with the rhythm of your breath.

Focus on drawing your belly into your backbone as you exhale, deeply and fully.

Pause as you feel the power of belly to back. Relax into the sensations.

Inhale again. Relax. Release.

Notice what you notice about how you feel in your body…

See how simple it can be?

By Cynthia Lynne, Lifeforce© Yoga Therapist   Copyright 2013

THE ESSENTIAL FOUR ELEMENTS OF TRANSFORMATION

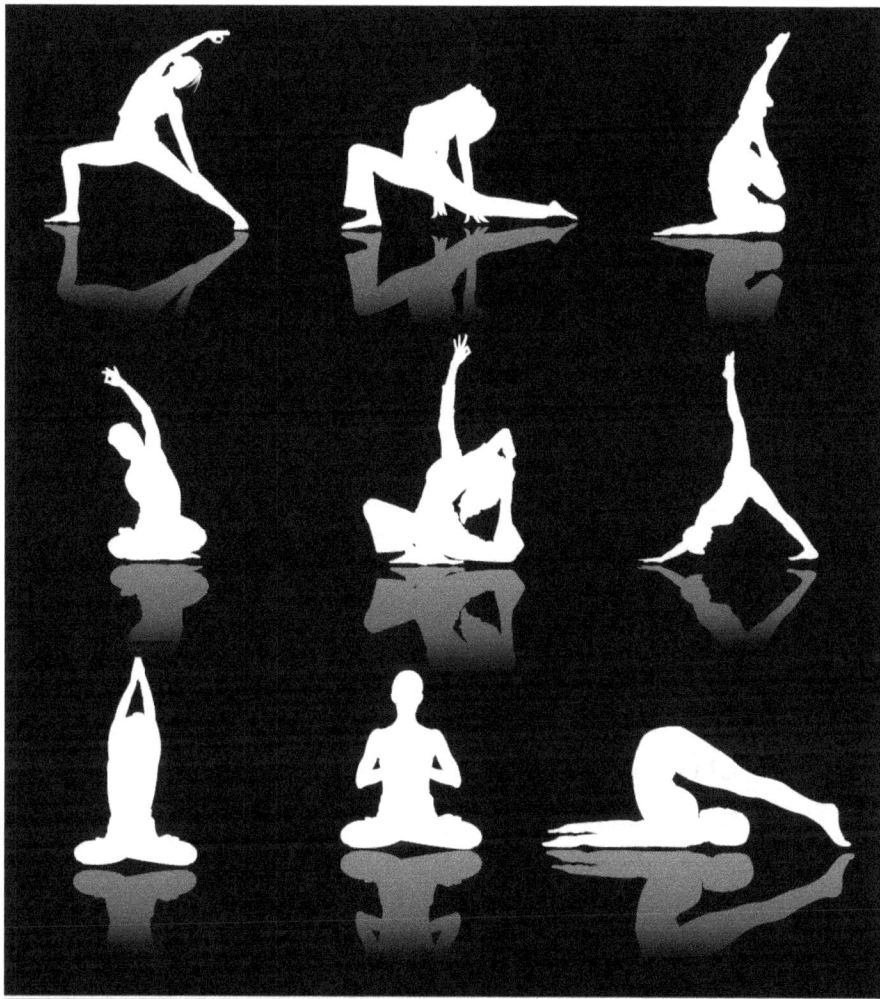

PATANJALI'S YOGA PRESCRIPTION FOR CHANGE

By Cynthia Lynne, Lifeforce© Yoga Therapist   Copyright 2013

DAILY PLANS OF YOGA ACTION

1. **ACTION :** Tapas is the Sanskrit word for "heat"
   The willingness to do whatever action is most necessary to reach a desired outcome.

2. **SELF STUDY/SELF AWARENESS**
   What you notice in response to your choices. Becoming present to who you are and who you wish to become to fulfill your divine purpose

3. **WILLINGNESS**
   To see truth for what it is which allows you to release the sufferings of illusions and self deceptions

4. **SET AN INTENTION** or a sankalpa:
   What action you will take to create your desired outcome.

Where is your Zen Zone?

THE ZEN ZONE :THE PLACE TO JUST BE

<u>Essential Commitment:</u>   "Hold Space " : Set Aside Time and Place

The Zen Zone – a place you create to discover the place within where calm strength resides.

The Zen Zone – peace from the inside out, the outside in…

Commit to create a place where you will be free from distractions and disturbances and other clutter.

Where in your home could you carve out this safe space? Where in your office? Where else could you be to feel completely safe?

This is your safe place to just BE. Do nothing more -- nothing less.

Dedicate this place for the practice of yoga.

Commit to holding this place for yoga and yoga only.

Use screens to partition space, add bolsters, pillows, rolled up blankets and mats.

Add candles, music, photos, a status of Buddha or Lakshmi – whatever inspires you into this place.

Become acquainted with the sound of stillness, the scent of lavender and the softness of a mat supporting a straight spine.

Get to know your self in a whole new way in the Zen Zone.

By Cynthia Lynne, Lifeforce© Yoga Therapist   Copyright 2013

ESSENTIAL YOGA : SITTING POSES

SITTING POSE: COBBLERS POSE   :   CROSS LEGGED POSE

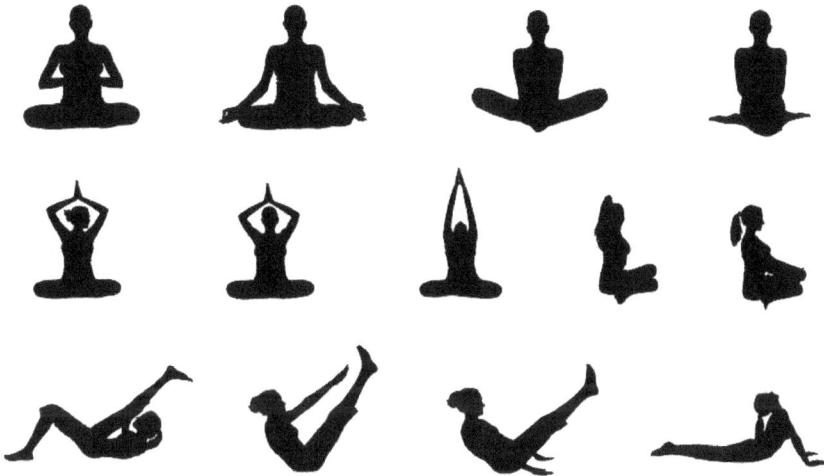

SITTING POSE with SUN SALUTATIONS   MODIFIED HEAD of COW
LEG STRETCH   BOAT POSE   SUPPORTED BOAT   COBRA

GUIDED PRACTICE : SITTING POSE SEQUENCE :

(1) Sit with you spine comfortably extended. (2) Roll your shoulders down and away from your ears. (3) Inhale and place the sides of your feet together; interlace fingers around toes and exhale as you gently stretch the groin muscles; use bolsters or blocks to support the knees without overextending into the stretch. (4) Cross your legs so that the right knee rests on the top of your left knee. Inhale deeply and as you exhale, gently stretch and release.

MODIFIED SITTING VOLCANO POSE: (middle)

(1) Raise your arms partially above the head, elbows slightly bent as you clasp hands together; shoulders down; turn head gently left, back to center, then right, back to center. (2) Extend arms fully; breathe deeply into your belly for three deep breathing patterns before you relax your neck as you gaze up towards your hands, palm to palm with fingertips outstretched

LEG STRETCH: (3rd line of poses)

(1) Lie on your back with your legs bent; feet flat on the floor. Be certain that your neck is comfortably supported; place a folded blanket beneath your neck to avoid strain: (2) Raise your right leg into a vertical position;
(3) Grasp with both hands, the right leg at either the calf or the ankle(do not overextend the leg; be certain your back remains flat on the floor; (4) Breathe deeply as you gently pull your leg towards your chest. Breathe deeply for a series of five complete breaths; focus your attention on the gentle stretching sensation in your hamstring.

THE BOAT:

(1) Breathe deeply and sit up; ensure that your sitting bones are adequately supported on the floor before you raise your legs and reach your arms towards your toes. (2) Inhale deeply as you bring your arms to the outside of your legs. Elongate the spine as you exhale and draw your navel towards your spine. (3) Grasp the backs of your thighs with your hands; inhale and lean back; balancing on your sitting bones. Breathe deeply for five complete breath rounds. (4) Release the pose; lower the legs slightly as your hands return to the floor. Breathe deeply five complete breath rounds.

COBRA POSE:

To prepare for the cobra pose, lie facedown with your forehead resting on the mat: Place your hands beneath your shoulders, palms down and elbows tucked next to the body. (1) Engage your abdominal muscles and feel your hip creases press into the floor. (2) Inhale, curl your upper body off the floor two to three inches as your slowly raise your forehead, nose, chin, shoulders and chest. Be certain your pelvis and hip bones remain flat against the floor. Shoulders are down and away from the ears. Keep elbows bent at a 45 degree angle or less. (3) Inhale deeply as you raise up slowly , keep your elbows bent and lengthen your neck. Hold the pose for 3-5 counts

Essential Yoga : Basic Sitting Poses

Begin by choosing a sitting pose – either half lotus or easy pose. Choose the pose that is most comfortable for you to sit supported with a straight spine so you can fully relax into your body.

EASY SITTING POSE

Sit on the floor with your legs in front of you.
Your spine is elongated.
Your arms rest by your sides. Shoulders are down away from the ears.

Cross your legs so that the arches of your feet are positioned beneath the outside of your calf muscles.

Your right foot should be under the left knee, the left foot under the right knee.

HALF LOTUS POSE

Follow instructions above for sitting with straight spine and comfortably supported sitting bones.

Place the sole of your right foot along the inside of your left thigh; turn the top of your left foot so that it lies on the top of your right thigh.
Be gentle with your knees and left ankle joint.

Place your hands gently on your knees with palms facing either up or down. Be certain the knees are supported by bolsters, blocks or folded blankets so that the knees are slightly higher than the hips.

Close your eyes or rest them half closed so that you can focus the attention on the rhythm of your breath.

Listen to the sound of your breath as your focus your attention on the ebb and the flow of breath in your body.

Settle in.

Feel the comfort of being safely supported by your spine as you relax fully into the support of a solid seated position.

ESSENTIAL DAILY YOGA PRACTICES : INTENTIONAL BREATH

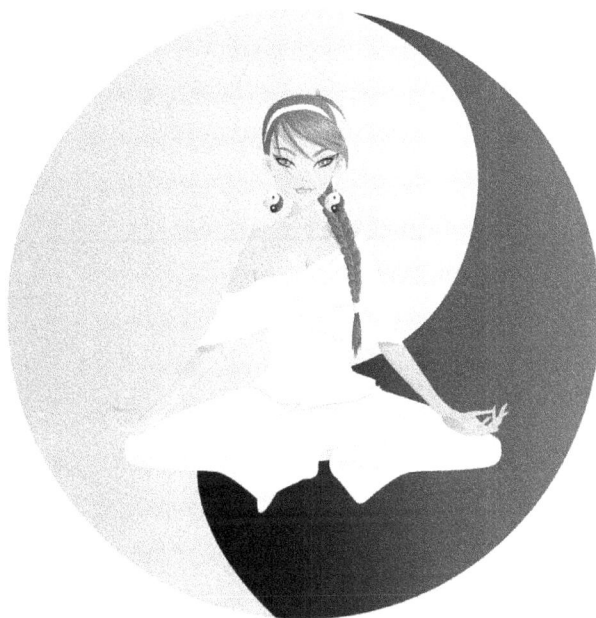

Integrated Sitting Poses & Intentional Breath Practices

By Cynthia Lynne, Lifeforce© Yoga Therapist   Copyright 2013

THE POWER OF INTENTIONAL YOGA BREATH PATTERNS

What if beyond simply noticing the rhythm of your breath, you could set an intentional breath pattern that would shift the energy in your body?

What if you could practice intentional breath patterns that would calm and quiet or energize and awaken?

What if your breath could become a tool to master stressors without losing clarity, focus or strength?

Intentional yoga breath patterns.

Discover the possibilities......

Mindful Body : Intentional Breath Patterns

Intentional Breath Practices are simple and powerful practices that will help you calm, energize and balance energies in the body and mind.

The patterns that follow are simple enough to start with and will give you an opportunity to experience the power of a simple patterned breath practice.

When you integrate breath patterns with flow sequences, you create a dynamic practice that breaks through any myths you may have that yoga is a static practice.

No, you don't need to buy an expensive gym membership, new tennis shoes or an outfit from LuluLemon.   You can get started in your home – or your office – any time you choose.

Commit and dedicate this place to your yoga practice.

Be amazed at what you will discover when you hold this space as essential.

CALMING BREATH
PATTERNS OF PRACTICE

Essential Breath Patterns: Focused Breath to Center & Align

As you inhale deeply into the diaphragm, draw the breath smoothly into the nostrils and focus all of your attention on the expansion of the exhaling breath.

Make it twice as long as the breath before.

As you exhale, notice where you most experience the sensations of relief and relaxation in your body.

Count ten of these deep breath beats.

Notice where you feel more relaxed in your body.
Is it your neck?   Is it your shoulders?

Notice how the breath has cleared space in the mind.
Breathe deeply, smoothly and slowly.

Notice your shoulders release the tightness as you relax into your breath.

Release the tension in your neck as your expand into your exhaling breath.

CALMING BREATH PATTERNS OF PRACTICE

ESSENTIAL CALMING BREATH PRACTICE : OCEAN SOUNDING BREATH

PURPOSE IN PRACTICE : This is a simple breathing pattern that will support you in gently relaxing the body and focusing the mind.   It is an excellent practice to start with on its own; as well as a simple practice to integrate in all pose and flow sequences.

MINDFUL BODY : SITTING POSE : Sit in your safe place, your spine upright, resting comfortably in your sitting bones; hips and knees supported by bolsters or rolled blankets.

Settle into a comfortable sitting position so that you can focus your attention inward. Allow all of your attention to rest of the sensation and rhythm of breath in your body.

MINDFUL BREATH AWARENESS : Notice the path of your breath as you inhale deeply in through your nostrils; your breath a thin thread of liquid light.

Pause as you slow the rhythm of your breath and focus on breathing deeper into your diaphragm as you draw in the next breath.

Draw into the thin liquid light of your breath. Feel the sensation of breath in your body.   Recall the ocean; remember the sensation of being at the beach. Notice if it is the sound or the smell of the ocean that you notice first.

Pause before you slowly exhale through the back of your throat into slightly parted lips.

SENSATE FOCUS : Listen to the sound of the breath as it moves into the nostrils, through the back of your throat as you exhale gently, releasing and relaxing as you tune in to deeper awareness.

MINDFUL RECALL : Recall the sound of water on the rocks as the tide ebbs and flows, bubbling and popping over the rocks, water and light as it ebbs and flows...the eternal rhythm of the ocean.

GUIDED PRACTICE : OCEAN SOUNDING BREATH ..continued

SENSATE FOCUS : Allow all of your attention to rest on the sound of breath you release into the sound of pebbles washed by the waves at the shore, as they ebb and flow, the water bubbles and pops as it rushes across the surfaces of the rocks…

INTENTIONAL BREATH : Breathe slowly. Smoothly. Deeply into the rhythm of the ocean tide. Like your breath, it has an eternal rhythm of its own….listen now to the sensations of breath deeper into your body. Let your self be in the rhythm of breath…ebbing and flowing…Become one with the sound of ocean, the sound of breath. I am one.

SUGGESTION FOR INTENTIONAL PRACTICE : Begin with 10 sets then gradually increase into 10 minute practice sessions. Integrate this breath into your yoga flow sequences to cleanse the body and mind. Integrate with music or ocean sound to fully absorb the body and mind in the sensation of release and relaxation.

ESSENTIAL CALMING BREATH PATTERN : SSSS

PURPOSE : This is a cooling breath practice to choose when you feel "wired" or physically agitated and "noisy" in your mind.

Inhale deeply into your nostrils, drawing the breath into the back of the throat.

Pause as you relax into the releasing breath.
Make an "S" sound through slightly pursed lips as you exhale.

Expand into the "SSS' sound throughout the length of the exhaling breath.

Pause. Relax. Remain suspended in this pause in between.

Reflect on the sensations of release and relaxation in your body,.
Inhale. Pause.

Expand your exhaling breath twice as long and relax .
Release deeply into your belly.

Notice the sensations of relaxation expanding into your belly center.
Relax.

Rest in reflection as you focus on the sensations you feel in your chest.
Notice the feelings of expansion and openness in your heart.

Practice the "sss" sound for up to five minutes;
Rest for an additional five minutes to focus on the sensations in body and mind.

By Cynthia Lynne, Lifeforce© Yoga Therapist   Copyright 2013

ESSENTIAL CALMING BREATH PRACTICE : LEFT NOSTRIL

PURPOSE : To target burn out symptoms of "agitated," "edgy," "wound up" or nervous and anxious.

PRACTICE : Do 10 sets of breath pattern: notice where you feel most calm – in your mind or in your body? Do another 10 sets to balance body and mind.

Sit in a comfortable position with your spine comfortably extended and supported.

Make a fist of your left hand. Next, release the thumb and the third and fourth fingers, keeping the index finger and middle finger folded toward the palm.

Close the right nostril with the fourth finger of the left hand.

Breathe in slowly and deeply through the left nostril.

Close the left nostril with the thumb and exhale slowly through the right nostril.

Focus on breathing deeply, smoothly and evenly.

Practice between ten and twenty repetitions before pausing.
Rest quietly in the sensations of relaxing into your body awareness.

ESSENTIAL CALMING & BALANCING BREATH PRACTICE   :
ALTERNATIVE NOSTRIL BREATH

PURPOSE : Nadi sodhana or alternate nostril breathing is an integrated
practice of both left and right nostril breathing. This breath practice brings
balance between calming and energizing.

PRACTICE : Start with 10 complete sets. Gradually increase to 10 minutes
of practice. Choose music to focus the mind while you immerse yourself in
the flow of your breath's rhythm..

Sit in a comfortable sitting pose of your choice, spine straight, shoulders
relaxed,

Breathe normally to clear nasal passages as you rest into the sitting bones.

To begin inhale through both nostrils, inhaling through the nostrils and
exhaling sharply through the nostrils – lips are slightly parted.

Close your eyes as you relax into a comfortable sitting position.

Start with the right hand; the second and third fingers rest on the bridge of
the nose for support. The remaining fingers are used to gently press the side
of the nose, alternately closing one nostril or the other.

Inhale through both nostrils.

Rest the thumb and ring fingers on your nose to gently close the right nostril.

Place your thumb on the right nostril; exhale slowly and evenly through the
left nostril; then inhale through the left nostril.

Inhale through the active nostril slowly and deeply. At the end of the
inhalation, close the active nostril, then slowly and completely exhale and
inhale through the passive nostril.

Repeat this cycle inhaling slowly through the open nostril, switching sides
after each complete breath cycle.

ENERGIZING BREATH
PATTERNS OF PRACTICE

MINDFULNESS BREATH ENERGIZING PATTERNS

GUIDED BREATH PRACTICE : RIGHT NOSTRIL VITALITY

<u>PURPOSE</u> : Choose this breath practice to lift the mood, release physical lethargy and energize the body and mind.

<u>PRACTICE</u> : Start your day with 10 sets of vitality breath ; take a breath break instead of loading up on sugary, caffeinated beverages

Sit in a comfortable position with your spine comfortably extended and supported.

Make a fist of your right hand.

Next, release the thumb and the third and fourth fingers, keeping the index finger and middle finger folded toward the palm.

Close the left nostril with the fourth finger of the right hand.

Breathe in through the right nostril.

Close the right nostril with the thumb and exhale through the left nostril.

Focus on making the inhale and exhale even.

Do between ten and twenty repetitions of this pattern.

Close your eyes and notice your energy.

If you feel too energized, practice a few rounds of Alternate Nostril Breathing to balance the energy.

MINDFUL BREATH PRACTICE : ENERGIZING
' BEE BREATH "

PURPOSE : This is a cleansing breath practice and deeply relaxes the body while calming the mind.   When feeling scattered, distracted or agitated, this breath practice will help you calm and focus into calm strength.

PRACTICE : Daily for 10 sets : Integrate into flow sequences at the end to fully clear the mind and release the body into calm strength.

Sit on the floor in a cross-legged position with your spine straight
Close your eyes and breathe deeply until you settle in comfortably resting in this pose.

After a full inhalation, begin making a gentle buzzing sound from the back of your throat as you slowly exhale. Imagine the sound of bees buzzing in a meadow of lush green grass and flowers the colors of rainbows reaching up to touch the sun.

As you exhale, feel the vibration of the sound rising out of the back of your throat, through the roof of your mouth and up into the brain.

Breathe deeply and smoothly into the sensations of relaxation you feel from head to toe.

Focus on the soothing sounds and sensations as they fill your body with a deep calmness; breathe slowly, smoothly and deeply. Let your attention become fully absorbed by the sensations within.

Inhale deeply into your belly as you release deeply into the exhaling breath;

Pause in the suspension between exhaling and inhaling. Allow your self to rest for a moment in these sensations.

Notice the sensation of pausing in the suspension between breath moments. Relax.

Breathe slowly, smoothly and deeply as you focus your attention on the sensations of deeper relaxation within your body. Notice the smooth rhythm of your breath as your body becomes absorbed by the sensations within.

Allow yourself to continue the practice up to five minutes.

By Cynthia Lynne, Lifeforce© Yoga Therapist   Copyright 2013

INTEGRATED BODY/MIND ENERGIZING PRACTICE

MINDFUL BREATH/BODY PRACTICE : PULLING PRANA

PURPOSE : This is a simple energizing breathing technique that stimulates the vagus nerve to support the body's release of endorphins, or "mood chemicals"   This practice is especially helpful if you feel depressed, lethargic or lack motivation.

PRACTICE : Do 10 sets of this practice ; begin and end your yoga flow sequences with this practice.

Stand with your feet a comfortable distance apart.   Or if you prefer a sitting position, settle into a comfortably supported spine.

Inhale deeply through your nostrils while extending your arms straight out in front of you with your fingers spread wide and your palms face up.

Make fists of your hands and vigorously draw them back to your waist with a forceful exhalation of breath through your nostrils.

Do this twenty times, then let your arms float to your sides.   Rest there and breathe quietly, deeply and slowly.   Feel the fullness of the energy throughout your body.

Close your eyes and breathe normally as you bathe in the effects of pranayama.

** This practice is adopted from Amy Weintraub's Yoga for Depression

HEALING THE BODY WITH MOVEMENT

By Cynthia Lynne, Lifeforce© Yoga Therapist   Copyright 2013

THE POWER OF A PURPOSEFUL POSE

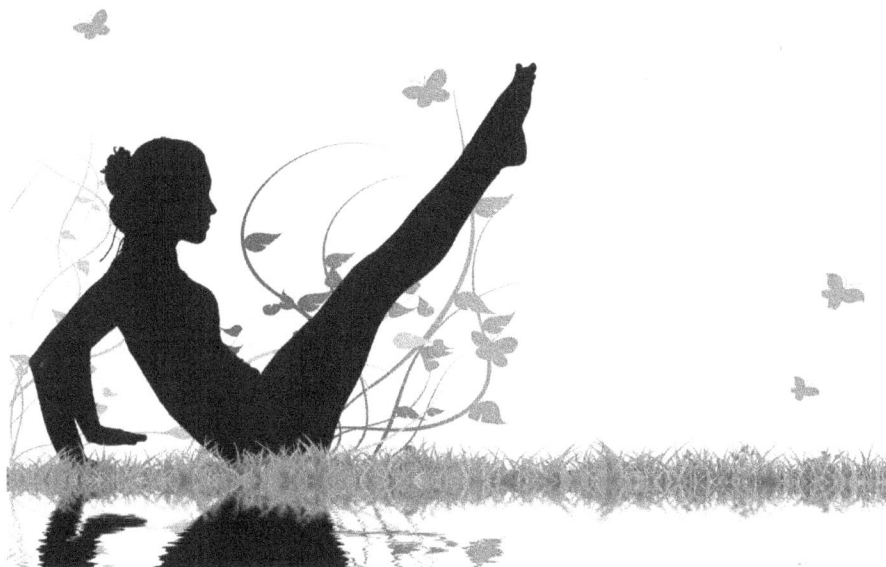

Let the power of the pose work for you in shifting the mind in the direction of your heart's most important desires.

Discover the power of a yoga warrior pose.
Align within the core of your feminine divine.

Awaken to your inner divine wisdom..

THE BODY AS A TEACHER

Changing beliefs....

What if listening to the wisdom of the body could set you free from the cycle of burn out?

What if your body could guide you into creative solutions for the problems your mind conjures up for you?

Would you be willing to listen?

Could you begin to believe your body is your ally – not an enemy to be conquered?

What one choice will you choose to start to do?

Consider the opportunities you could create when you let go of forcing yourself into an artificial change your mind dictates you into.

Instead, consider the possibility of going with the flow of yoga…

Learn to trust the power of a daily yoga practice to change the course of your thoughts, just as it will change the way you move in your body.

All you need to do is take a leap of faith….commit to a decisive action on behalf of transformation….

Why settle for a little bit of change…go for the bold!

Yoga Inspired Fitness Choices : What If You Chose....

    (1) Strength Builders Fitness Choice:
       Action Steps to Initiate Change :

    (2) Endurance Builder Fitness Choice :
       Action Steps to Initiate Change:

    (3) Balance Builders Fitness Choice:
       Action Steps to Initiate Change:

    (4) Flexibility Builders Fitness Choice:
       Action Steps to Initiate Change:

    (5) Grace Builders Fitness Choice:
       Action Steps to Initiate Change:

By Cynthia Lynne, Lifeforce© Yoga Therapist   Copyright 2013

THE ESSENTIAL STRETCH :

MINDFUL PRACTICE SUGGESTION :
Practice each of the following poses individually, then link them together in a flow sequence for a simple morning practice.

BASIC STANDING POSES : MOUNTAIN POSE

PURPOSE : *Mountain pose is a fundamental pose providing proper alignment for other standing poses. Anchor in the strength of being fully supported by your stance, like a roots of a tree are supported by mother earth.*

Stand tall with your spine straight , with legs hip width apart and feet parallel.

Place half of your weight onto the heels of your foot; the other half on the balls of your feet.   Feel your big toes pressing down into the earth.

Allow the thighbones to move towards the hamstring muscles in the back of your legs. Feel the knee caps lift. Feel yourself lifting out of the waist.

Notice how it feels when your shoulders are relaxed and your chin is level with the floor.

Hunch your shoulders up towards your ear lobes then down again to stretch out and relax the tension gathered in the shoulder and neck area.

Inhale deeply, filling the lungs slowly and smoothly,. Keep your arms by your sides, stretching your fingertips towards the floor.

Exhale deeply as you fully relax your shoulders; feel the strength as the energy runs from head to shoulder to elbow to fingertip, to elbow to shoulder, to chest, into the belly and down into the tips of your toes.

Take ten deep breaths to feel the fullness of increased energy and strength.

Raise your arms overhead with palms facing one another; Relax your shoulders down as you stretch your spine into the fullness of the mountain pose. Notice the deep sense of calmness you feel as you rest in this quiet strength.

MOUNTAIN POSE WITH EXPANSIVE BREATH

PURPOSE : Integrate deep breathing into the strength of a fully supported mountain pose feeling the power of being anchored in and fully supported by your body..

Stand with your feet shoulder width apart. Hold your arms straight out in front of you with palms together at chest height.

Be certain your shoulders are down and away from the ear lobes.

Inhale through an open mouth as you throw your arms open and back,, bending the wrists so your fingertips point away from you..

Lift the chin slightly and your eyes look upward.

Exhale completely through the mouth as you begin to come forward, tucking your chin, slightly bending at the waist and knees.

Hands may be clasped together in the front of the chest or they may right on your thighs.

Let your head hang so that there is no pressure on your neck.

Relax into the release of your spine holding your neck as you release deeper into the rhythm of your breath.

Inhale deeply as you raise up, slowly, vertebrae by vertebrae.

Move your arms back again to the extended (not hyperextended) arm position as you exhale deeply through the back of your throat, making a "hhhhhaaaaa" sound as you relax.

Let your arms remain extended out to the sides, stretch your fingertips; notice the strength of your arms as you lower them slightly, three degrees down before returning to the extended position. Breathe deeply for five breath beats before repeating the pattern five more times.

ESSENTIAL YOGA WARM UP : TORSO TWIST

PURPOSE : *This stretch loosens the arms, torso, spine and waist. This poses energizes your upper body and allows you to release tension and tightness from sitting too long.*

Stand with your feet shoulder width apart. Let your spine be comfortably extended, your shoulder away from the ears.

Let your arms hang loosely by your sides.

Engage the abdominal muscles slightly,.

Begin turning your upper body, shoulder first, from one side to the other.

As you alternate, allow your arms to swing slowly as though they were empty coat sleeves.

Let your head follow the movement of your upper body,.

As you pick up the pace, allow the heel of your right foot to come off the floor when your body turns to the left, your left heels rises slightly when your body turns to the right,

Repeat this side to side motion for ten complete torso turns (one=left to right; right to left)

Gradually slow the motion until you return to the center. Breathe deeply into your diaphragm and exhale slowly and deeply.

Feel the stream of light energy throughout your body as you take time for ten patterned breath counts of your choosing.

ESSENTIAL YOGA WARM UP : STANDING ON TOES

PURPOSE : *This pose strengthens the calf muscles, stretches the soles of the feet and massages the balls of the feet. It helps with balance and increases concentration*

Stand in mountain pose with arms by your sides.

As you inhale, raise your heels from the floor, rising up onto the balls of your feet.

Exhale slowly and deeply as you come back down.

Repeat this movement for five breath beats.

Inhale and rise once again onto the balls of your feet, bring your arms up, raising them above your head.

Remain on your toes with your arms raised for five breath beats.

Return your feet to the floor and your arms to your sides.

Repeat five times.

Notice the feelings of strength in the calf muscles; feel the power of increased balance and concentration.

ESSENTIAL YOGA WARM UP :
SUPPORTED FORWARD BEND

PURPOSE : *This pose lengthens and aligns the spine, reduces lower back pain and helps keep the back and neck flexible. The backs of the legs and hamstring muscles are also stretched. In addition to relaxing the body, this pose also increases circulation and can relieve fatigue. You may find that using the wall for support allows you to let go and relax into the stretch for a deeper experience.*

Stand about a foot away from a wall.

Elongate the spine and be certain your feet are hip distance apart.

Let your buttocks rest against the wall.

Bend slightly forward, hinging at the hips. Bend your knees slightly.

Reach around and use your hands to lift the flesh of the buttocks up and away from the sitting bones.

Bend your arms and grasp your elbows with your hands. Allow your head to hang loosely between your bent arms.

With each exhalation breath, let your body relax a little more. As you inhale, lift ever so slightly and then release gently into the exhale, relaxing the head into the arms further.

Breathe deeply for five deep breath beats.

Straighten the arms. On the next inhaling breath, slowly begin to come up, one vertebrae at a time,.

Elevate your chin from your chest to make sure the head comes up last and there is no strain on the neck or back.

ESSENTIAL YOGA WARM UP : PALMING

PURPOSE : *This is a practice that both energizes and relaxes at the same time. Try this in a comfortable sitting position. Sit comfortably with your spine supported in an upright position.*

Begin by rubbing your palms together for about fifteen seconds until you generate heat.

Then, without putting any pressure on the eyes, press on your brow and on the cheeks outside the bony rims of your eye sockets.

Feel the sensations of warmth from your palms as you breathe gently into your cupped hands.

Continue to keep your chest upright but allow your head to gently tip slightly backward as you focus your attention in on the rhythm of your breath.

Notice the color and texture of any visual patterns beneath your hands

Allow those images to fade into black as the muscle of your face release and relax.

Focus your attention on the gentle rhythm of the ebb and flow of your breath and the sensations of muscles in your neck or shoulder relaxing as you let go of any tension or tightness preventing you from feeling peace.

ESSENTIAL YOGA WARM UP : TAPPING

PURPOSE : *This practice promotes energy restoration; releases shoulder &*
neck tension as well as negative emotional energy.

Tapping these three meridien points releases tension from the body.

(1) Cup your hand and tap the center of your collarbone
with a rapid, circular motion for 15 seconds.

(2) Next tap the shoulder in the same way for 15 seconds;

(3) Next tap the side of the rib cage.

(4) Rest as you breathe deeply; notice the sensations of
relaxation and warmth in your body.

(5) Repeat the exercise for 5-7 minutes; tapping for 15
seconds, then resting for 15 seconds.   Repeat on the
other side of the body.

ESSENTIAL YOGA WARM UP: YOGA MUDRA

PURPOSE : This pose loosens the shoulders, arms and spinal column; it improves posture and back problems.

Stand with your feet parallel, hip width apart.

Clasp your hands behind you, interlacing the fingers.
(If your shoulders are tight, hold a strap between your hands.)

Bend your knees, tuck your chin toward you check and lower into a forward bend,.

With your hands still clasped, allow your arms to fall forward up over your lower or upper back without straining.

Breathe deeply, slowly and rhythmically as you hold the pose for five counts.

On an inhalation breath, begin to raise your upper body, keeping your knees slightly bent,

Slowly raise your chin. Your head comes up last.

Breathe deeply as you return to the upright position.

Release your hands slowly, letting your arms float back to the sides of your body.

Feel the release of tension in your neck, shoulders and back.

ESSENTIAL YOGA FLOW

Yoga Flow Sequences

ESSENTIAL DAILY PRACTICE :
SUN SALUTATIONS

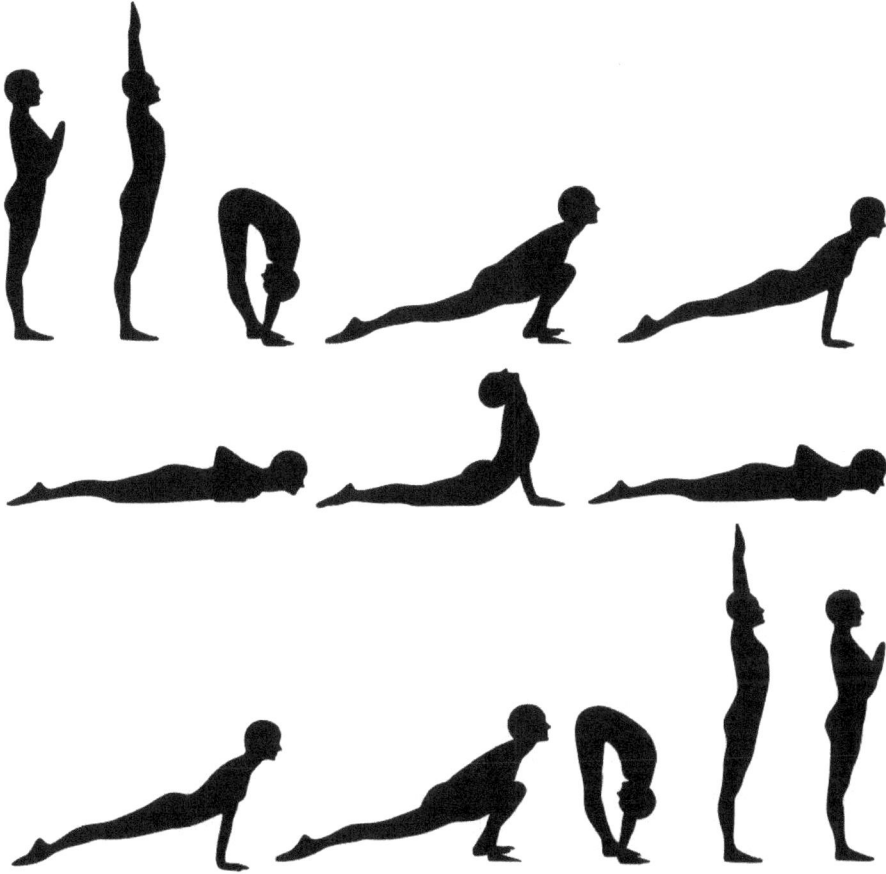

GUIDED SUN SALUTATION FLOW SEQUENCE

SUN SALUTATIONS :
THE POWER OF PRACTICE

Sun salutations are used to warm or energize the body. This introductory flow sequences warms the body for more challenging poses that follow. It can be a flow sequence within itself.

Sun salutation is a graceful sequences of poses executed as a continuous, flowing motion. The poses are linked with the breath. Each asana counterbalances the one before, stretching the body and elongating the spine forward and backward. These movements expand and contract the chest to regulate breathing.

Focus your attention on moving in and out of center; extending away from center and drawing back into center as you connect more deeply to your core. Awaken both strength and fluidity in the abdominal and pelvic muscles are you drawn your mind and breath into your vital center. Allow your mind to return its focus to the center of your body throughout the practice.

Allow the movement of your body to follow your breath rather than tailoring your breath to every movement. Follow the lead of your body through breath and centering your focus on the vital center.

Sun salutations can be an intentional meditation to connect with the inner light and the sun's energies that bring us the essence of life's force energy

Visualize the sun as it spills warmth and color into the morning skies. Recall the sensations of the sun warming your skin as you breathe deeply into the feelings of energy moving throughout your body; energizing and calming you at the same time.

Guided Sun Salutation Flow Sequence:

(1)Stand in Mountain Pose with feet parallel: Hold your hands in front of your chest with palms together in Namaste.   Inhale fully and deeply; exhale slowly and deeply

(2) Inhale and lift your arms over your head, with palms facing but not touching. Bend upper torso back slightly.

(3)Exhale and bend forward at the waist into a Forward Bend, tuck your chin towards your chest and bend your knees slightly.

(4) Inhale and extend your left leg straight behind you into Kneeling Lunge; your knee, shin and toes rest on the floor; your right foot is forward between your hands with the knee over the ankle.

(5) Exhale and bring your right leg back. Support the weight of your body on your hands and toes; Inhale into a "push up" position, engage and tighten your thighs and abdominal muscles; be sure your back is supported by the floor.

(6) Exhale and lower your knees, thighs and upper chest to the floor

(7) Inhale and lower your hips and raise your upper torso into a Cobra, keep your shoulders down and your pelvis pressed down towards the floor:

(8) Exhale and raise your hips into downward dog.

(9) Inhale; step your left foot between your hands; extend your right leg straight behind you, your knee, shin and toes rest on the floor;

(10) Exhale; bring the right foot forward; bend down at the waist with palms resting on the floor; or knees bent slightly if you cannot touch the floor

(11) Inhale and raise up by engaging the abdominal muscles, lifting the chin and keeping the knees slightly bent; Raise the arms overhead with palms facing but not touching. Bend the upper torso back slightly.

(12) Exhale and bring hands in front of your heart in the Namaste position. Inhale and exhale fully and completely.   Repeat all twelve steps; bring your right leg backward at step 4.

ESSENTIAL RESTORATIVE YOGA

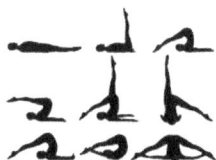

YOGA FLOW SEQUENCES

RESTORATIVE YOGA : DEEP RELAXATION POSE

PURPOSE : *To deeply relax body and mind ; can be used as a preparation for yoga nidra. When the pose is done by lying back over a bolster, the rib cage expands naturally so that you breathe more deeply, more slowly . Yogis find this pose to be energizing due to the effects of the slight backbend but also restful.*

This pose is an excellent pose to use between poses and at the end of a yoga session. Resting in this pose allows the body and mind to fully absorb the positive effects of your poses or flow sequences.

The position of the head is crucial in Savasana and other restorative yoga poses.

If the chin is elevated relative to the forehead, the position will be stimulating.

When the chin is even with the forehead or slightly lower, it is easier to relax.

If necessary to achieve the desired angle of chin, elevate the head with a pillow or folded blanket .

RESTORATIVE YOGA POSE : Savasana

On a yoga mat with blankets or bolsters to support the knees and neck as needed to fully rest in a reclining position.

 Lie flat on your back with your arms by your sides, palms up.

Keep your legs about a foot apart.   If you feel discomfort in the small of your back, place a bolster or rolled blanket under your knees.

Close your eyes.

Breathe deeply and slowly into your belly.

As your breath slows and deepens, notice the release of the tension your body has been holding and notice the sensations of sinking deeply into your yoga mat.

As you relax more deeply into the pose, simply notice your breath.

Let go of the need to control your breath with your mind.   Let your mind focus all of your attention on the sensations of relaxing into the rhythm of breath in body.

Rest in this pose for ten minutes.

When you come out of the pose, bend your knees into your chest; roll over onto your side while your eyes remain closed.

Remain on your side for a moment or two before you use your arms to slowly push yourself to s sitting position, bringing your head up last

.

ESSENTIAL RESTORATIVE YOGA :
LEGS UP THE WALL

Set up for the pose by placing a bolster or a stack fo folded blankets parallel to the wall and approximately six inches away from it.

You may need to adjust the prop farther from the wall if your hamstring muscles are tight. To come into the pose, wiggle up to the wall and sit on and to one side of the bolster.

Place your hands on either side of the bolster and swing your legs up the wall.

If you are on a bolster, your tailbone should rest just over the front edge of the bolster so that your sacrum(triangular bone at the base of your spine) angles down toward the floor. This maintains the normal inward curve of your lower spine and makes the pose more relaxing.

Rest comfortably in this pose for five minutes or longer.

By Cynthia Lynne, Lifeforce© Yoga Therapist   Copyright 2013

ESSENTIAL RESTORATIVE YOGA : CHILD'S POSE

In your safe place, kneel with the buttocks on or near the heels.

Bend from the hips, stretching the upper body out, forward and down onto your thighs.

Rest the forehead on the floor or on a rolled up blanket so that you can relax fully in to the resting pose.

Let your shoulders round and relax as you breathe deeply into the body.

Relax as you allow your breathing to become slow and deep, at least five full deep patterned breaths.

MINDFUL MEDITATIONS :

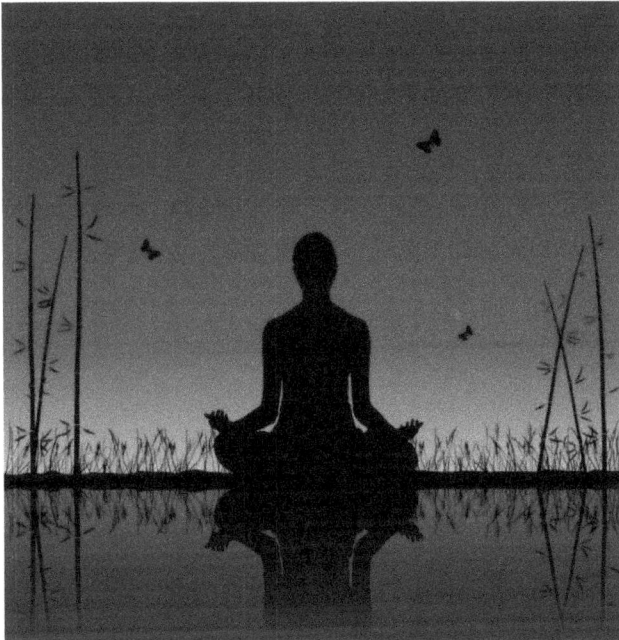

COURTING PRESENCE OF MIND

By Cynthia Lynne, Lifeforce© Yoga Therapist   Copyright 2013

MINDFULNESS MEDITATIONS : BECOME PRESENT

Mindfulness meditation practices help you train your mind to better concentrate and relax.

Mindfulness meditation helps your brain expand into creative, resourceful states of accelerated problem solving.

When you become mindful and present within this moment in time, you are shifting your consciousness from an active state of doing, to a state of reflecting more deeply into the sensory awarenesses of this moment in time.

===

THE MIRACLE OF MINDFULNESS MEDITATION PRACTICES

Herbert Benson was often startled and amazed by benefits of meditation practices he saw in his studies throughout the world.

He witnessed Tibetan monks dressed in nothing but loincloths, wrapping themselves in wet sheets in freezing temperatures at 15,000 feet in the Himalayas. Instead of shivering, dropping their body temperatures and potentially freezing, the monks visualized fires in their bellies, raising their body temperatures enough to dry the wet sheets.

===

===

COURTING PRESENCE : IN THE MOMENT :

Simply notice the fullness of the moment you are in by engaging with all five of your senses.

What is the color of the room you are in?
What does this place look like?
What does it sound like?
What is the scent of this moment in time?
What is the texture of the present moment?
How does it taste if you were to savor the flavor of the moment?

GUIDED IMAGERY

Create a focal point of awareness for the mind to rest within. Let your mind create a picture or "mind movies" of a serene scene, a peaceful place or another image you can absorb yourself within.

Begin with simple mindful inquiries, such as:

Where do you choose to rest your mind?

A soft cushion? A fluffy cloud? The mirrored surface of a placid pond?

You could choose to rest your attention on an image of a serene nature scene while quiet music plays in the background of a lavender scented room.

MINDFUL FITNESS CIRCUIT TRAINING EXERCISE

Begin by sitting in a comfortably supported position that allows you to be relaxed yet alert at the same time.

Focus on resting the mind. If you like, visualize the breath to be a quiet resting place or a cushion or a soft pillow where your mind can rest comfortably. Breathe deeply as you rest in the sensations of releasing and relaxing.

FOCUSED ATTENTION : Begin to shift into focused attention. Bring your fully attention to the rhythm of breath – or any other focal point of awareness you choose. Let this attention be steady as a rock, undisturbed by any distractions.

As your attention begins to wander, gently and firmly bring it back to this resting place again and again. Breathe deeply into your body and notice where your body releases tension and tightness in the shoulders or neck or back. Rest comfortably in this state of awareness for several moments.

OPEN ATTENTION : Next shift into open attention. Bring your attention to whatever thoughts, feelings or sensations arise in body and mind. Let this attention be flexible like grass shifting with the winds.

In this mind there is no such thing as a distraction. Every object you experience is an object of meditation. Continue to rest in this state of awareness for several moments more, breathing deeply and comfortably into your body. Shift to focused attention for three more minutes.Then shift to open attention for three more minutes.

COMPLETE THE MEDITATION CIRCUIT: Begin to complete this exercise by focusing your attention once again into a resting place, a cushion, a soft pillow. Let your mind rest here in this place of calm strength. Relax fully until your body is ready to return to a state of calm alertness.

Take a few moments to shift gradually into full alertness. Focus your attention on the sounds of being in the present, the color of the room you're in and the texture of the floor beneath your feet.

By Cynthia Lynne, Lifeforce© Yoga Therapist   Copyright 2013

MINDFULNESS PRACTICE EXERCISES :

===

EYE FIXATION TECHNIQUES :

Choose a point on the wall opposite or a candle or a softly lit lamp.

You could also choose to hold a pen at arm's length and use this as a focusing point.

Or you could choose a mandala, focus your attention on the bindu(center dot) and the colors and patterns of art designed to heal.

GUIDED PRACTICE :

Rest in your sitting pose until you are settled in to a straight spine and fully supported back. Breathe deeply. Notice your shoulders relax. Breathe.

Rest your gaze on your chosen focal point of deepening awareness. Allow your gaze to settle in as you continue to relax into your body's calm center.

Breathe smoothly, slowly and deeply to find your strength there. As your eyes close completely or rest half closed, allow your mind to become completely absorbed within the rhythm of breath as you rest in the picture your mind holds safe for you.

MINDFUL MEDITATIONS : IMAGERY & NATURE

<u>Mindful Imagery</u> : Recall a favorite place in nature. A forest. A meadow. A mountain scene.

<u>Mindful Inquiry</u>: What do I feel in my body when I remember my serene scene? Is it the image of the mountain standing majestic in its strength?

<u>Intentional Breath</u> : Breathe deeply as you contemplate this sensation. Focus your attention on the ebb and flow of breath in your body. Relax into breath and expand into your center.

<u>Mindful Inquiry</u> : Is it the pine scented breeze that gently lifts the hair off your neck? Breathe into the scent of the mountain that brings you closer to this place.

<u>Mindful Sensations</u> : Is it the warmth of the sun on your skin as you walk through the lush green meadows embraced by the mountain's rocky peaks? Breathe and you recall the sensation of sun warmed skin.

<u>Mindful Sounds</u> : Is it the sound of the water rushing against the rocky creek bed as you walk deeper into the valleys just the other side of the meadow? Breathe deeply into your body as you remember.

<u>Mindful Imagery</u> : See your self walking through the mountain pass twisting up towards the summit.

<u>Mindful Reflection</u>: Notice it feels different to be embraced within the center of the mountain, different than when you were at her feet, looking up.

MOUNTAIN MEDITATION …. Continued

Intentional Breath : Breathe quietly as you notice the sensations through your body.

Mindful Viewpoint : Now, see your self moving towards the mountain peak. : Notice when you have reached the peak of the mountain. See your self standing there.

Mindful Sensate Focus : Breathe slowly, smoothly and deeply. Expand into your exhalations until you feel centered within your body.
Rest your attention on the rise and fall of your belly as you relax fully into this awareness for at least one minute, if not two.
Relax. Notice now how it feels when you are atop the mountain. Feel the strength throughout your body as you stand tall.   Breathe deeply into the feeling of earth and air.

Mindful Reflections: Mindful Distinctions : Notice how it feels different to be atop the mountain. Look around. To the right. To the left. Back to the center.   Breathe quietly into your body. Feel the sensations throughout your body like waves of lavender light throughout your body.   Feel the sensations in your body as you breathe deeply into the center of your mountain strength.   Release and relax into the power of tranquility.   Feel the sensations warm throughout your body as you breathe quietly.

Mindful Sensate Focus : Absorb the sensations as you absorb the warmth of the sun on your skin.   Be present to the power of these sensations in your body. Notice the sense of calm strength you experience within body and mind as you notice these sensations of calm strength throughout your body.

Bring with you this strength as you begin to return to a greater state of alertness. Breathe fully into the calm strength you feel throughout your body.

MINDFUL MIND CLEARING MEDITATION :

<u>Mindful Inquiry</u> : What if negative thoughts are like the clouds that sometimes drift by the mountain?

<u>Mindful Reflection</u> : Contemplate how solid and stable the mountain is throughout the changing seasons.

At times the mountain may be clouded over, its peaks covered in fog.

Other times the mountain is assaulted with thunder and lightning and torrential rains.

Sometimes the mountain rises into a crystal clear blue sky, awash in sunshine.

Throughout rain or sleet or snow, whatever the changing seasons bring, the majestic mountain stands steady and strong,

What if you too, could stand like the majestic mountain, steady and strong, undisturbed inside.

Let mindful awareness be unwavering and steady – like the mountain

<u>Intentional Breath</u> : Breathe deeply and smoothly; notice the even rhythm of your breath, feel the sensations rise and fall in your body.

Relax. Sit quietly breathly deeply, slowly and smoothly.
Feel the sensations of strength and peace

<u>Mindful Sensate Focus</u> : You *can* remain steady and strong inside. Feel the power of your quiet strength. Notice it now. Breathe slowly, smoothly and deeply into the center of your body. Let go there. Now. Breathe.

MOUNTAIN SKY LAKE MEDITATION :

This can be a meditation in and of itself – or it can be integrated with the above meditation.

<u>Mindful Imagery</u> : As you stand strong in mountain pose, visualize a scene of a majestic mountain range. Take time to feel the grandeur of majestic peaks reaching up towards the sky as you stand at the foot of the mountain.

<u>Mindful Sensate Focus</u> : Feel the coolness of the shade, the breeze as you breath deeply into the scent of cool green pine and moist earth beneath your feet.

Notice how tall the mountains stretch into the limitless blue sky, does the mountain touch the sky – or does the sky touch the mountain?

Contemplate this mystery as you breathe deeply into the luminescent blue of the limitless sky.

Let your attention move away from the mountain peaks to the crystal clear lakes the Himalayans call "sky lakes" because they so perfectly reflect the sky above.

Protected by the rocky mountain peaks and trees, the surface of the lake is smooth and calm.

Reflect on the lake and notice how it reflects the light and sky.

Notice how perfectly the sky lake mirrors the soft blue of the sky above.

Notice how transculent the turquoise blue waters are; notice how you can see into their depths.

<u>Mindful Breath</u> : Let yourself breathe deeply into your body. Let your mind become as clear and smooth as the surface of the pond; focus your attention on the smoothness of your breath as you relax more deeply into your body.

MINDFUL MEDITATIONS : SKY LAKE REFLECTIONS

<u>Mindful Reflections</u> : Let your attention rest on the surface of the translucent blue water. Notice how it is like a mirror. See how you can see your face and the sky above on its surface.

As you imagine yourself looking into the surface of the water, notice how the water reflects only what is there, neither editing out nor adding in.

The water reflects the stormy darkness of the stormy clouds the same as the wispy white clouds drifting across the blue sky. They are the same.

Imagine your mind is as translucent and reflective as the sky lake.

<u>Mindful Intentional Breath</u> : Breathe deeply into the feeling of expanding into your exhaling breath.

Let your body rest in this awareness,   Reflect upon its truth while you notice the calmness you feel without your body.

You release attachments with each breath you take.

Breathe in as you see yourself as the water of the sky lake, breathe out, reflect.

Pause in the suspension between this time and space and feel the power of being present.

Notice how it feels to be inside the picture while you picture the picture. Rest in contrasting awarenesses.

How does it feel to see the picture?
How does it feel to be inside the picture you see?

MINDFULNESS MEDITATIONS & MANTRAS

MINDFULNESS MEDITATION : NAMAHA

PURPOSE : *Namaha is a Sanskrit word which means "not me" or "it is not about me." This simple meditation provides a powerful focus that calms and soothes the worried mind, releasing the body from internalized emotional stress. Integrating meditation and mantra/sounding is a powerful way of healing the body and mind at a profound level. Practice these practices up to ten minutes.*

PRACTICE: *Daily: Integrate into morning and/or evening practice.*

SIT QUIETLY: Sit comfortably in a quiet place where your spine is comfortably straight, your legs crossed in a sitting lotus pose or hero's pose if you prefer. Focus your attention on the rhythm of your breath.

BREATHE:

INHALE: Breathe slowly and deeply in through your nostrils

PAUSE slightly before you release into the exhalation:

EXHALE: slowly, deeply from the back of your throat through slightly parted lips.

PAUSE slightly as you remain "suspended" in breath awareness before you begin the pattern again.

INHALE: Begin again, drawing your breath deeply from the center of your body as if drawing water from a well.

REPEAT SILENTLY as you

PAUSE: It is not about me. Namaha.

EXHALE: ,slowly, deeply and smoothly from the diaphragm.

Notice the sensations of relaxing as you release into the truth of namaha.

INHALE: REPEAT SILENTLY: All is well. Namaha

PAUSE: REPEAT SILENTLY: There is a greater plan. Namaha.

EXHALE: slowly and deeply, feel the tension unravel as you relax fully into this exhaling breath:

PAUSE: REPEAT SILENTLY: I have faith. Namaha.

SIT QUIETLY: Remain resting in this energy and light until you are ready to awaken fully feeling deeply refreshed and restored.

ESSENTIAL MINDFULNESS MEDITATION :
CIRCLE OF LIGHT integrated with SO HAM MANTRA

PURPOSE : *This practice will develop your concentration, clarity and inner stability by providing a single object as a focal point of awareness. Practice daily integrating with either a.m. or p.m. practice. Start with ten minutes and gradually increase to twenty to thirty minutes or more.*

PRACTICE *:* Sit on a chair or cross legged on the floor with a cushion or a folded blanket under your hips., Use enough support to lift the hip joints slightly higher than the knees.

VISUALIZE : Close your eyes; mentally draw a circle of light around yourself. Allow yourself to clearly visualize a circle that separates you from the world of daily life – both the outer world of perception, and the inner world of patterns preoccupations and habituated thinking patterns. Set the intention to now see yourself sitting inside this circle of light.

Notice how it delineates a space within which you can hold your awareness. Notice how safe and protected you feel from disturbances and distractions. Notice the feeling of resting the entire body as you sit comfortably still, release any unnecessary tightness or tension; pay attention to the movement of your breath.

INTENTIONAL BREATH : Refine your awareness as you focus on the rhythm of your breath as it becomes smoother, more subtle, deeper and longer. Focus on the sensations in your body as you release and relax into the exhaling breath.

SENSATE FOCUS : Notice how the energy moves from your heart throughout your limbs as you inhale again, smoothly, deeply from the center as you relax into the exhaling breath, feel the energy flow back into the center of your chest, then down more deeply into your diaphragm as you exhale once again.

INTEGRATE SOUND : Next practice inhaling while saying "so" and exhaling into the "ham." Take time to practice this until you are comfortably aligned with the rhythm of breath and mantra.

A PERFECT YOGA FIT

CUSTOM DESIGNED PRACTICE SEQUENCES

Create a personalized yoga plan of daily action that inspires you!

Begin a daily practice to discover the practice your body will fall in love with....

Court your heart's desires by listening as you begin...

What yoga pose inspires you into strength, power and passion?

What yoga pose lifts you into the spirit of dance?

By Cynthia Lynne, Lifeforce© Yoga Therapist   Copyright 2013

CUSTOM DESIGNED YOGA SEQUENCES
Prescriptions for Healing & Awakening

SITTING POSE SEQUENCES

Align with Intuition with sitting yoga practices
    a. Sitting Lotus with Patterned Breath Sequences (centering, aligning)
    b. Ocean Breath, (calming, soothing, relaxing)
    c. Alternate Nostril, (balancing both energies)
    d. Namaha (calming mind, soothing body)

Align with body with energizing prana
    a. Breath of Fire
    b. Pulling Prana
    c. Right nostril breath

==

STANDING POSES

==

Awaken body and mind with powerful poses and flow
sequences

      a.   Sun Salutations (energizing flow)
      b.   Restorative Yoga Practice (calming flow)
      c.   Pulling Prana (energizing)
      d.   So Ham (calming and centering)

==

====================================

5 INSPIRED YOGA FLOW SEQUENCE PRACTICES

====================================

a.FIVE ESSENTIAL SITTING POSES :

Half lotus, seated hero, turtle, bound angle and boat   (calming , centering and anchoring)

b.FIVE ESSENTIAL RECLINING POSES :

Restorative yoga poses; including child's pose and corpse (calming, soothing and relaxing) : cobra, reclining spinal twist, knee hug

c.FIVE ESSENTIAL STRETCHING POSES :

Eagle, neck rolls, shoulder shrugs, expansive and kneeling yoga mudra (physical release and relaxation)

====================================

==

ESSENTIAL YOGA FLOW SEQUENCES : FOR MORNING & EVENING PRACTICE

Awaken, energize and balance mood with:

1. <u>Morning Practice Flow Sequence</u>: Sun Salutations (awakening, energizing)

2. <u>Evening Practice Flow Sequence</u>: Moon Salutations (calming, releasing, relaxing)

3. <u>Standing Poses:</u> Mountain Poses with Expansive Breath, Torso Twist, Downward to Upward Dog (anchoring, grounding, energizing)

==

A MINDFUL JOURNAL GUIDE :

From YOGA DESIGNS : A MINDFUL JOURNAL GUIDE

START WITH THE END IN MIND :
THE POWER OF PURPOSE

If you could choose to be the creator of your life options rather than a victim to your burn out, what else would you choose?

What inspires you?

Why not reflect upon your mindful possibilities while your body eases into new yoga possibility poses…

MAKE POSSIBLE THE IMPOSSIBLE :

Is it possible? When you believe it is, it is!

What would it take for you to believe…
   In the power of transformation?
   In the power of the breakthrough moment?
   In the power of ….YOU?

What if you chose to set your self up for success?

What successes could you immediately create for yourself?
What would the power be in your being present?

What if … you could start with a different outcome in mind….
What would you like your better outcome to be?

What if it becomes even more possible when you allow your
imagination to vision your future possibilities for you?

Take a moment to picture it in your mind…

THE FREEDOM TO BE : EXERCISE YOUR RIGHT TO CHOOSE

The freedom to choose.   The freedom to be.

It's your choice…isn't it?

You *are* free to choose what you decide. You are free to change your mind.

You are free to simply be rather than constantly do, do, do….

Why not choose to let go of burn out beliefs and court the opposite?

You are free to choose changing your mind with mindfulness, aren't you?

One tiny choice, one radical transformation.

SUCCESS STRATEGIES :

Create Results Oriented Action Statements:

Your mindful mind can become your new best friend. Focus your mind into the Zone of Genius and be amazed at who you are and what you can create!

Focus on the result you most desire to create – this is only slightly different from setting goals in that you are actually envisioning the result you want to create rather than simply stating a goal.   State the result as if it is happening in this present moment:

For examples:
Results oriented focus: I focus on a daily yoga flow practice that includes 3 variations of warrior to build strength and endurance.

Results oriented focus: I master all three balancing poses so I can hold the poses for three minutes each. Or: I will develop endurance by holding poses for two minute interval

Results oriented focus: I listen to yoga nidra with the restorative yoga sequence I practice a to relax into a more restful sleep.

MINDFUL INQUIRY : GAINING CLARITY

Settle in to your Zen Zone with a Journal, find your Zen Center and relax deeply into presence before asking the following questions :

WHAT I MOST WANT TO CREATE FOR MY FUTURE :

MY BIGGEST ROADBLOCK IN ACHIEVING THIS THUSFAR HAS BEEN:

HOW DO BURN OUT MINDSETS/BELIEF SYSTEMS FEED INTO THIS PROBLEM?

WHAT ARE MY PRIMARY BURN OUT PATTERNS/ HABITS

HOW WOULD IT BE DIFFERENT IF I WERE FREE FROM BURN OUT?

WHAT I COULD CREATE IF I WERE FREE FROM BURN OUT BELIEFS, HABITS OR PATTERNS?

Essential Priority Commitments: What are yours?

MINDFUL INQUIRY : *If I believe in not only change but transformative change, what would I most desire to change in the above referenced beliefs, habits or patterns?*

Set at least three and up to five essential priorities that you will focus all of your attention and energy into achieving:

Write your desires as results oriented statements, focus on your desired outcome:

(1)

(2)

(3)

(4)

(5)

THE POWER OF PURPOSEFUL INTENTIONS

Start with the end in mind …see how you succeed…

Say what you'll do to make the change you most desire to create.
Write it down.

See it in your mind's eye.
Become fully immersed in the picture of your success.

Commit to it. Promise you'll keep your promise.
Say what you'll do. Do what you say.

Support the power of the imagination to focus forward.

Let mind and body co-create your new vision of powerful possibility.

Committed Decision : Committed Action

Be a committed decision taker – what change do you wish to step in to NOW, in this present moment in time?

INFINITE POSSIBILITIES ....
IF YOU KNEW…

If you knew beyond all doubt… you could *get twice as much done in half the time*, would you take ten minutes a day to meditate?

If you knew beyond any and all uncertainties… you could *remain calm in the face of any storm*, would you take ten minutes a day to do yoga?

If you knew…you too, could be calm strength…you, too, *could be laser focused*, would you take ten minutes now to practice?

THE TRUE NATURE OF CHANGE

Transformation is a force of nature….not a change to be forced by an unnatural thought, idea or belief adopted long ago to protect or provide something no longer needed

Align within the forces of nature to transform beyond any change you could presently imagine…

Shed outdated belief systems….

Turn your attention inward…

Listen for the wisdom of the body to rise up and guide you…

Be inspired by how powerful you can become when you are motivated by deep and true desire!

Discover the infinite possibilities of mindfulness by moving into mindfulness now!

By Cynthia Lynne, Lifeforce© Yoga Therapist   Copyright 2013

==

YOGA TRANSFORMATIONS : A MINDFUL NEW BEGINNING truly is a beginning!

Once you fall in yoga love, it's good to know there's more love to grow into, isn't it? To deepen and expand the power of your yoga transformations, check out the creative resources available to guide into your source of infinite wisdom:

YOGA DESIGNS : MINDFUL JOURNAL WORKBOOK:

Discovery journal to guide you deeper into your custom designed yoga practices.

YOGA TRANSFORMATIONS : A MINDFUL NEW BEGINNING : Audio Program

YOGA TRANSFORMATIONS:TWENTYONE DAYS TO TRANSFORM COACHING PROGRAM

Everything you need to get past "I don't have the willpower" blocks. *Transform in body, mind and spirit with your own at-home practice and laser focused coaching to keep you on path and accountable to your imminent success!*

ZEN CENTERED WOMEN'S LEADERSHIP RETREATS

Visit www.cindynaughton.com for more information on our yoga inspired coaching programs and retreat intensives for women thought leaders and enterprising entrepreneurs.

==